VIRUS DISEASES AND
VIRUSES

CAMBRIDGE
UNIVERSITY PRESS

University Printing House, Cambridge CB2 8BS, United Kingdom

Published in the United States of America by Cambridge University Press, New York

Cambridge University Press is part of the University of Cambridge.

It furthers the University's mission by disseminating knowledge in the pursuit of education, learning and research at the highest international levels of excellence.

www.cambridge.org
Information on this title: www.cambridge.org/9781107659568

© Cambridge University Press 1938

First published 1938
First paperback edition 2014

A catalogue record for this publication is available from the British Library

ISBN 978-1-107-65956-8 Paperback

VIRUS DISEASES AND VIRUSES

BY

SIR PATRICK P. LAIDLAW

M.A., B.Ch., F.R.C.P., F.R.S.

THE REDE LECTURE
1938

CAMBRIDGE
AT THE UNIVERSITY PRESS
1938

VIRUS DISEASES AND VIRUSES

The study of virus diseases and viruses is one of comparatively recent date, and yet in the course of the last few years it has become of outstanding interest to all biologists and many biochemists. Knowledge regarding this group of disease agents commenced in 1894, when Iwanowski showed that the disease of tobacco plants known as "mosaic disease" could be transmitted by an agent which would pass through the pores of filters which were sufficiently fine to hold back all ordinary bacteria. In 1898 Beijerinck, independently, discovered anew the filterability of the infecting principle of tobacco-mosaic disease and wrote of a *contagium vivum fluidum* as the cause of this disorder. This conception, which was contrary to accepted doctrine at that time, has not been destroyed with the growth of knowledge, but has, more recently, owing to Stanley's work with the same disease agent, gained in strength. In 1898, again, Loeffler and Frosch showed that the virus of foot-and-mouth disease of cattle would pass through filters which were impervious to bacteria and that the disease could be transmitted in series from animal to animal by means of what appeared to be sterile filtrates. With these striking examples of disease, induced by agents which were apparently differentiated from bacteria by their minute size, it is not a little remarkable that recognition of the importance of viruses should have been delayed for so long, and it is perhaps the more remarkable since the early workers foresaw clearly the possible applications of their new knowledge to other diseases. However, if advance in the study of virus diseases was slow to commence with, it has proceeded with an ever-increasing acceleration, until to-day it has become exceedingly difficult to keep abreast with the advances which are made almost daily. There are still just a few workers who are sceptical regarding the existence of viruses and who endeavour to explain the essential experimental results in other ways, such as, for example, filterable forms of ordinary bacteria. But the number of the unbelievers is small and steadily diminishing. The great majority of competent observers recognise that a special group of agents called viruses can cause many diseases in man, animals, plants and even in bacteria themselves. These diseases are of great importance and the sum total of the disharmony they produce rivals that caused by the visible bacteria.

In the case of man we now know that many of the acute infectious fevers are caused by these peculiar agents, as for example small-pox, measles and mumps, and probably chicken-pox. Each of these is responsible for much suffering, though the first-named is now, for us, of smaller importance owing to the introduction of Jennerian vaccination in 1796, long before the nature of the causative agent was appreciated. Warts, *Herpes febrilis*, epidemic influenza, yellow fever, infantile paralysis and some forms of encephalitis are all caused by viruses. Only those who have seen many cases of infantile paralysis can realise the damage it may cause to a population or the disability from partial paralysis which may be left behind on recovery from the acute stages of the disease. Yellow fever, once the most dreaded infectious disease of the tropics, is still a severe threat to the well-being of man in many parts of the world, but the pioneer work of Walter Reed and his co-workers, who proved that the infecting agent was filterable and transmitted by mosquitoes, did much to assist in combating the ravages of the disease. An intensive anti-mosquito campaign instituted by Surgeon-General Gorgas enabled him to rid Havana of yellow fever for the first time for many years. Subsequently, by still more strenuous efforts on a wider front, he eliminated yellow fever completely from the Panama Canal zone and reduced the incidence of malaria to quite small figures. This allowed the completion of the great waterway between the Pacific and the Atlantic. Stokes, Bauer and Hudson showed that the virus could be transmitted to rhesus monkeys, and this led to an intensive study of the malady on an experimental basis. These studies cost the lives of some of the workers. Adrian Stokes did not live to see even the first-fruits of his discovery, and Noguchi and Young also died from the disease. Many who have worked with yellow fever have contracted the ailment, but now, thanks to much experimental work, we know of methods of immunisation which can be employed to protect laboratory workers and others exposed to infection. The methods are not easy to apply on a really large scale and yellow fever still remains to a large extent uncontrolled.

Typhus fever is included in the group of virus diseases by some authorities and excluded by others. Typhus is not now common in civilised communities, but it was once one of the greater epidemic scourges of mankind. It flourishes where large numbers of people are herded together under insanitary conditions, such as have obtained during military campaigns. Zinnser, in his very interesting book, *Rats, Lice and History*, shows how important this disease has been in the past, how it has influenced crusades and interrupted wars. He states: "It is hardly debatable that the power of Napoleon in Europe was broken by disease more effectively than by military opposition or even by Trafalgar." And one of the more important diseases which ravaged Napoleon's armies was typhus fever. During the Great War typhus caused serious trouble in Russia and the eastern front, but very fortunately the western front escaped this deadly ailment, though that comparatively trivial kindred disorder known as "trench fever" was common enough.

To quote Zinnser once more: "The establishment of the Haitian Republic, though usually attributed to the genius of Toussaint l'Ouverture, was actually brought about by yellow fever. In 1801 Napoleon sent General Leclerc with 25,000 men to Haiti to put down the revolt of the Negroes. The French troops landed at Cap Français, defeated Toussaint, and drove him into the interior. The Negro army was rallied and reorganised by Dessalines, but could not have

(9)

successfully opposed the well-disciplined and well-equipped French troops had not an epidemic of yellow fever disorganized the invader. Of 25,000 Frenchmen, 22,000 died. There were only 3000 left to evacuate the Island in 1803."

Animals and birds suffer from virus diseases as commonly as man, and some of the disorders are of considerable economic importance. Swine fever and "hog-flu" have proved to be great sources of worry in pig ranches where large numbers of swine are herded together, and they are still sources of trouble, though not quite so serious, to those who keep pigs in small groups. Swine influenza is a particularly interesting example, because Shope proved that this disease was caused by the combined attack of a virus and a small haemophilic bacillus. Later Andrewes, Smith and myself, and Shope and Francis, showed that the virus element in this disease, though distinct, has close relationships with the virus of human epidemic influenza; moreover the human and porcine diseases show certain striking resemblances. Louping-ill of sheep, a tick-borne disease, causes much worry and loss to the sheep farmers in Scotland. It can infect other species, including man, but apart from its natural host, the sheep, it rarely causes serious trouble. South African horse-sickness and equine encephalomyelitis, the latter another insect-borne disease, may be the cause of much anxiety and loss for the horse owner. Rabies is another example, but this is of little importance to Great Britain thanks to the rigid quarantine laws for imported dogs. Dog distemper, besides taking toll of many young dogs, is now recognised as a serious menace to the fur farmers, for silver-foxes, mink and fitches may suffer severely from the disease. The losses from virus diseases are greater when the affected animal population is crowded together, and this condition frequently obtains in fur farms when large numbers of susceptible young animals are coming to maturity. Three widespread outbreaks of dog distemper swept over Greenland in 1888, 1896 and 1904, with the result that sledge transport by dogs was seriously interfered with and this caused great hardship to the human inhabitants.

Foot-and-mouth disease, which is historically interesting, is also a disease of great economic importance, as is well illustrated by the experience on the continent during the latter half of last year. Foot-and-mouth disease is due to a very small virus (one of the smallest known), and this commonly infects cattle, sheep, pigs and goats, though a number of other species are also susceptible. The disease is an acute infectious fever characterised by a vesicular eruption in the mouth and on the feet. The mortality from the virus disease alone in the adult animal is not high, though young animals suffer much more severely and serious losses may occur in young stock; but, as is often the case with virus infections, complications are common, and in this instance these may include the loss of a hoof, spreading septic infection up one or more limbs, local gangrene and occasionally pneumonia. From these complications losses are often very considerable. Even if no complications develop, the convalescent animal takes a long time to recover and regain a condition which will satisfy the farmer. Contact infection is easy to understand, but the precise mode of spread of this disease to remote places is not understood, and control has proved exceedingly difficult. In this country the disease is notifiable, and whenever an outbreak occurs which is confirmed by a Veterinary Inspector of the Ministry of Agriculture the whole of the affected herd is slaughtered and the carcasses burnt. Disinfection is undertaken and limitations regarding the movement of animals in the neighbourhood of an outbreak are imposed for a time, while a careful watch is kept for any sign of further disease in the district. Put quite briefly, whenever this disease gains access to this country it is eliminated by a slaughter policy and compensation is paid to the farmer for the animals destroyed. In the greater part of the continent of Europe the slaughter policy is not in force, and attempts are made to control the disease in other ways. In 1936 there were a few sporadic outbreaks of foot-and-mouth disease on the continent and such as did occur did not spread to any significant extent. In May 1937 the disease broke out in the south of France, apparently introduced by sheep imported from Algeria, and gradually spread all over France, to Switzerland, Belgium, Holland and Germany. By the end of 1937 there had been at least 130,000 outbreaks in France, 63,000 in Belgium, 100,000 in Holland and 36,000 in Germany. Each of these outbreaks involved considerable numbers of animals, so that the total of cattle involved during the year must have been very large. With a disease of this type spreading so freely and widely on the continent it was impossible that Great Britain should escape, but thanks to the watchful eye of the Ministry of Agriculture and its officials, together with the loyal co-operation of the farming community, the total outbreaks in this country up to the end of the year only reached 187. The epizootic was not over by the end of the year, but it is abundantly clear that it has cost the continent several million pounds and this sum is likely to increase, while Great Britain has suffered comparatively slightly.

Birds show many interesting examples of virus diseases, such as fowl plague, fowl-pox, pigeon-pox, canary-pox and infective laryngotracheitis, but there is one group of outstanding interest at the present time and that is the group of filterable viruses which were originally shown by Rous to be associated with the production of tumours indistinguishable from true sarcomata. In recent years there has been much work inspired by Rous's observations on fowl tumours, designed to explore the possibility that cancers in animals might be due to viruses. It cannot be said that any mammalian cancer has been shown to be associated constantly with, or caused by, a virus, but there is evidence from the work of Rous with the Shope papilloma virus and that of Andrewes, Ahlström, Gye and Foulds with the Shope fibroma virus that viruses may play some part in the production of malignant neoplasms. The work is in its infancy and what the ultimate outcome may be cannot be foretold, but the investigation is at a very interesting stage at the moment.

Psittacosis or parrot fever also deserves special mention, as it is exceedingly infectious, can cause a severe disease in man, and is one of the largest of the filterable viruses.

The virus diseases of plants are not only of great theoretical interest but many of them are of immense economic importance. A few appear to cause very little damage to their hosts. The variegation in colour of certain flowers such as "Tulip-break" is caused by a virus, and a similar condition in self-coloured stocks and violas was shown by K. Smith to be due to a similar cause. Many of the mosaic diseases are much more serious. The classical tobacco mosaic, for example, does a great deal of damage to infected plants and this has serious results for the growers, but it is almost impossible to obtain reliable figures on which to assess the loss to the industry caused by this virus. In the case of sugar-cane mosaic some figures are available. Coons shows that in Louisiana alone the introduction of disease-resistant varieties of sugar-cane raised the yield of sugar from 1636 lb. to 2440 lb. per acre, an increase of approximately 50 per cent, and he calculates the annual benefit obtained from the resistant strains on 250,000 acres at 5,975,000 dollars. The gain is mainly, but not entirely, due to resistance to virus infection, and when we remember that the figures given apply only to one small area, and that wherever it is grown sugar-cane is subject to mosaic disease, the aggregate world loss due to virus must be enormous.

Again, for "curly-top" virus of sugar-beet, Coons points out that, in California, the introduction of partially resistant varieties led to an overall gain of $2\frac{1}{2}$ to 3 (short) tons per acre, and this is estimated to give a financial benefit, on 102,000 acres, of 1,657,000 dollars.

In England the deterioration of local potato stocks and the poor quality of local "seed" potatoes is largely due to their contamination with viruses. The introduction from Scotland of "seed" potatoes, which are normally comparatively free from virus, raises the crop yield by about one ton per acre. As there are about 500,000 acres in England and Wales planted annually with potatoes, of which about 380,000 acres are planted with local "seed", the annual loss to the country from potato virus disease may be estimated to be about two million pounds.

When plant viruses are applied to the intact surface of healthy plants they are unable, in the majority of instances, to infect the plant. To effect an entry they require the assistance of some minor surface injury, and in nature many viruses are known to be transmitted by particular insect vectors. Some of these vectors, having fed once upon a virus diseased plant, remain infective for the rest of their lives. As K. Smith points out, this suggests that the virus multiplies in the body of the insect. The observations are strikingly similar to those recorded for the mosquito vector of yellow fever in the case of man. Once infected this mosquito is infected for life and there is direct experimental evidence that the virus multiplies in the body of this insect. The successful control of yellow fever by means of adequate anti-mosquito measures suggests that some plant viruses might be controlled by an attack on the appropriate insect vector, but so far there has been very little success in this direction. Nevertheless, the study of vectors of plant viruses is very important. The freedom of Scotch "seed" potatoes from virus is very largely due to the scarcity or absence of the appropriate vector (*Myzus persicae*) in the "seed"-growing areas of Scotland.

The bacteriophages form another important group of virus–disease agents. These were originally discovered by Twort (1915) and have, since then, been extensively studied by d'Herelle and many others. They possess the property of in-

fecting and multiplying in young growing bacteria, which they ultimately dissolve or lyse. Like
other viruses they will only infect particular species
and will only multiply within a living host. A
single species of bacterium may be attacked by
very many different bacteriophages, and thus the
number of species of bacteriophage is exceedingly
great.

The virus diseases which have been referred to
are merely a few representative examples out of
the very large number which might have been
mentioned—a full catalogue would only have
been wearisome—and everyone will agree that
the examples mentioned form a very remarkable
collection. Indeed, the collection of diseases con-
tains such varied and diverse elements that it is
not obvious why they should be classed together
in one group. The justification for the grouping
lies in the peculiar properties of the infecting agent
which causes the disease in each case. All viruses
are infective agents of small size; they are all at
the verge, or below the limits, of visibility by
ordinary microscopic methods and are sometimes,
on that account, called "ultramicroscopic". The
infective agent will pass through filters with pores
sufficiently small to hold back all ordinary pathogenic bacteria and for that reason they have been

called "filterable". Thirdly, viruses cannot be cultivated apart from susceptible living cells. Inside the cells of living organisms, or in tissue cultures, viruses multiply with astonishing rapidity, but when isolated from living cells they have never been shown to have any detectable metabolism.

These three negative characters are now insisted upon by the orthodox before an infective agent can be included in the virus group, but if we apply this ruling with rigidity classification of certain infectious agents becomes very difficult. For example, the organism associated with pleuro-pneumonia of cattle can be cultivated on ordinary laboratory culture media, and it is, on that account, excluded from the true viruses; yet this organism is filterable, has forms on the limits of resolution by the ordinary microscope, and had it not been cultivated it would probably still be regarded as a typical virus. Or again, what appears to be a minute cocco-bacillus (*Rickettsia prowazeki*) has been demonstrated in typhus-fever infections and shown to be correlated with the transmission of disease in lice and animals. On that account certain authorities would exclude typhus from the list of true viruses, and it is very doubtful if such exclusion is justifiable. With closer study and improvement of methods of examination small structures have been proved to be associated with other virus infections, as for example, vaccinia and psittacosis, but they have not yet been excluded from the virus group. However, if the distinction between the smaller pathogenic bacteria and the larger viruses is difficult, there is no doubt as to the classification of the great majority of the members.

Besides the three cardinal features which we have mentioned, there are others which are common to numbers of viruses but inconstant for the whole series. Most of the viruses withstand the action of 50 per cent glycerine better than the majority of bacteria; many are resistant to the action of carbolic acid or other chemical agents, yet the findings applicable to many are not constant for all. Certain viruses give rise to "inclusion bodies" within the cells which they infect; yet such structures are often limited to one particular type of cell in a given virus disease and in many virus diseases inclusion bodies have never been demonstrated. In certain instances inclusion bodies appear to be small masses of degeneration products within infected cells, but in others they appear to consist of aggregations of the virus itself, as for example in ectromelia, or in the case of the crystalline inclusions found in plants suffering from tobacco-mosaic disease. Most viruses can withstand drying, and the majority can be preserved in the dry state for long periods of time. In the case of birds and mammals, recovery from a virus disease is frequently associated with an immune state which lasts for many years, for example, on recovery from yellow fever or measles, man appears to be immune for life; a similar state of affairs obtains with rinderpest in cattle, swine fever in pigs and distemper in dogs. The immune state is frequently more solid and durable than is met with in the case of bacterial diseases, but the distinction is not constant, as is shown by influenza, the common cold or herpes, in man, where one attack does not protect against a second or third. In plants, where no humoral immunity has been demonstrated the virus usually persists in the host for life. The immunity is of the non-sterilising type and is, on the whole, inferior to that found in animals.

At one time it was considered that viruses had very rigid limitations as to the species they were capable of infecting, and though it is still true that they show very distinct preferences in this respect, yet the more viruses are studied, whether in plants or animals, the less rigid the species limitation is found to be. Viruses can be forced upon animals they do not normally infect—for example, human influenza can be made to grow in mice—or they can be induced to grow upon a particular tissue in an unsual host—yellow fever and South African horse-sickness can now be propagated in the brains of mice. These examples, and others might be quoted, show that viruses can still adapt themselves to changes of environment. It is true that the adaptation is limited owing to the obligate parasitic habit of the viruses, but it is none the less observable. Moreover, the adaptation to a new environment is sometimes accompanied by other changes in the virus itself, increased infectivity for one species may be, but is not always, associated with fall in virulence for another. Such changes when they occur may be of great practical significance—neurotropic strains of yellow fever and South African horse-sickness viruses can be used with comparative safety in the immunisation of men and horses respectively where the original virus would be too dangerous. The several members of the group vary considerably in this power of adaptation to new species and modification of character. It would seem that some viruses are unstable species and prone to variation, while others are more rigidly confined to a constant type.

Goodpasture and Woodruff showed in 1931 that certain viruses would multiply on the chorio-allantoic membrane of the developing hen's egg, and it has been shown since by Burnet and others that this structure is unusually receptive for viruses, even for many which will not infect the adult bird, and with certain limitations the fertile hen's egg is proving to be a very valuable subject for virus studies. Unfortunately there are a few viruses which will not grow on this structure, including the two important members, the virus of polio-myelitis and that of foot-and-mouth disease.

Mammalian viruses can also be grown in tissue cultures, either in minute fragments of tissue nourished in plasma and embryo extract, or by the more simple technique of utilising the sparser growth which occurs when minced embryo tissue is incubated in Tyrode solution. This simplified technique is proving to be of increasing utility in virus studies, and Li and Rivers have shown that it is possible to prepare bacteriologically sterile vaccinia, in quantity and as efficient as calf lymph, suitable for the prophylactic vaccination of human beings. It is interesting to note that plant viruses may also be propagated serially in root-tip cul-tures, but so far the tissue cultures of plant viruses are principally of academic interest. Salaman has, however, recently shown that potato virus "Y" may undergo attenuation when grown in root cultures of tobacco plants. Prolonged serial sub-culture of mammalian viruses on egg membranes or in tissue culture has been shown in some instances to lead to modification of the properties of the original virus and it may become relatively avirulent for the parent species, but in most instances the characters of the viruses remain unchanged even after prolonged serial passage. Egg-membrane culture and tissue culture are particularly useful when the virus under study causes the appearance of characteristic cell changes, such as the production of inclusion bodies. But there are many instances where no diagnostic cell change occurs and then recourse must be made to experimental animals or plants, for in the end our only criterion for the existence of a virus is the disease it induces in a susceptible species.

It will be realised that the study of viruses is beset with difficulties and usually demands a large equipment, but the difficulties, though manifold, have not been allowed to stand in the way of the study of this very important and interesting group of disease agents. They are of such immense significance for the well-being of man, animals and plants that every effort must be made to endeavour to prevent or control the ravages they may cause. Time does not permit us to consider the many interesting chapters which have been written on the prevention and control of virus disease.

But apart from the utilitarian aspects, the virus diseases offer fascinating problems to the biologist, such as what is the smallest form of living matter and what is the irreducible minimum of a parasite capable of transmitting a disease? What, in fact, are viruses?

If we try to summarise what we have reviewed so briefly we find that viruses appear to be very small obligate parasites, and within the limitation imposed by strict parasitism they show growth, multiplication, adaptation to environment and minor variations. These features suggest that the viruses are merely minute parasitic organisms, but there are certain difficulties in the way of accepting this view.

Studies in the last twenty years have shown that though all viruses are small, some are much smaller than others, and there is a very wide range in size between the largest and the smallest members of the group. A consideration of what we know regarding the range of size will give us a better appreciation of the great virus problem, namely, what a virus really is.

There are a number of viruses on the verge of visibility by ordinary microscopic methods. In the case of vaccinia, for example, the disease is always associated with very large numbers of re-fractile granules which can be stained by intensive methods; by deposition of stain upon the surface the apparent size of the granules is increased. Minute bodies were described by J. Buist as long ago as 1886 as occurring in vaccinia and in small-pox, but his observations appear to have been overlooked until recently. They were, however, described again by others, notably by Paschen in 1906, who maintained till his death that they were the causal agent of the disease. They are now sometimes known as Paschen bodies, or under the more general name of "elementary bodies", because similar granules have been seen in association with many other virus diseases. With ordinary visual light, whether by transmitted or dark ground illumination, it is not possible to obtain an accurate estimate of the size of such small objects, so recourse was made to photomicrography using ultraviolet light, for by the use of these shorter wave-lengths it is possible to secure critical photo-graphic images of objects which are too small to be resolved properly with visual light. In this direction Barnard has done much valuable work and he has been able to measure the sizes of some of the larger viruses with precision and to form fair estimates of the sizes of some others.

Filtration experiments have also given much valuable information regarding the sizes of viruses. In the earlier work, which established the existence of viruses, the filters employed were made from diatomaceous earth (Berkefeld) or from unglazed earthenware (Pasteur-Chamberland), and though these were usually efficient in separating the viruses from bacteria they could not be graded into degrees of fineness with any great accuracy; moreover, the mass of the filtering material was a serious drawback and caused errors from adsorption of the virus on the very large porous mass of the filter itself. However, with all their drawbacks, these old filters are still used extensively for many types of work. In the determination of size of viruses a great advance was made by Elford when he devised a method for making thin, tough, collodion membranes with fairly uniform pores and showed that, by slight alterations in the conditions of manufacture of the membrane, the pore-size could be varied at will. With a complete series of membranes graded according to the sizes of their pores, a rich suspension of virus and suitable test objects it is possible to determine the size of any virus with considerable accuracy—we have only to determine which size of pore lets the virus through freely and which size just retains all the virus. When a virus suspension is filtered successively through membranes of descending pore-size, infective filtrates of nearly uniform potency are obtained down the series until shortly before the limiting pore-size for the virus in question is reached, when there is an abrupt fall in the infectivity of the filtrate. With membranes having a pore-size only slightly less than this, inactive filtrates are regularly obtained. The data seem to show that each virus has its own characteristic size of particle and that in a virus suspension all the particles are of approximately the same size.

Collodion membranes can be used to purify and concentrate virus suspensions or to separate a small virus from a mixture of small and larger, as was shown by K. Smith, who has used membranes of this type extensively in his studies of plant viruses.

The centrifuge and the ultracentrifuge have also been used to estimate the sizes of virus particles, to concentrate them and to purify them, and some of the results obtained will be referred to later. Here we may note that the information as to the sizes of virus particles calculated from centrifugation data agrees with the results obtained in filtration experiments with "Gradocol" membranes. Again, in the case of the larger viruses, the sizes as established from ultraviolet light photomicrographs harmonise with the filtration figures. There are some minor discrepancies between the sizes as determined by the different methods, but it must be remembered that the calculations from filtration and centrifugation experiments are based on the assumption that all virus particles are spherical, and this assumption cannot be justified. However, these discrepancies in the estimate of the size of any one virus are trivial compared with the great variation in size which exists between the larger and the smaller viruses, and it is fair to conclude that the approximate size of the infecting agent in many virus diseases is now established within fairly narrow limits.

Some of the information regarding the sizes of a number of representative viruses is summarised in the table on pp. 30–31. It has been compiled from data largely supplied by my colleague Elford, and shows the sizes of some of the smallest free-living bacteria, various representatives of the group of viruses we are considering, and a few protein molecules. It will be observed that the range of size is very large, from about one-quarter of a

From Micro-Organism to Molecule

Table showing the diameters, in millimicrons, ot some micro-organisms, representative viruses and some protein molecules.

Name	Diameter
Chromobacterium prodigiosum	750 mμ.
Spirillum parvum	350 mμ.
Psittacosis virus	250 mμ.
Spirochaeta pallida Agalactia of goats and sheep	200 mμ.
Organism of bovine pleuropneumonia Sewage micro-organisms A, B, C Vaccinia virus Canary-pox virus Rabbit fibroma virus	150 mμ.
Rabies virus Infectious ectromelia virus of mice Herpes virus Pseudo-rabies virus	125 mμ.
Influenza virus—human and porcine Borna disease virus Newcastle disease of fowls	100 mμ.
Vesicular stomatitis virus	85 mμ.

Name	Diameter
Rous sarcoma virus Fowl plague virus Potato virus X	75 mμ.
Bacteriophages Staph. K, C 16, D 4, D 12	60 mμ.
Bacteriophages D 54, S 41, megatherium	35 mμ.
Rift Valley fever virus Equine encephalomyelitis virus Papilloma virus of rabbits	30 mμ.
Tobacco mosaic virus St Louis encephalitis virus Bacteriophages T 111, C 36, D 13, D 20, D 48	25 mμ.
Haemocyanin (Helix)	24 mμ.
Yellow fever virus	22 mμ.
Louping-ill virus of sheep	17 mμ.
Poliomyelitis virus Foot-and-mouth disease virus of cattle Bacteriophage S 13	10 mμ.
Edestin	8 mμ.
Serum globulin	6·5 mμ.
Serum albumin Oxyhaemoglobin	5 mμ.
Egg albumin	4 mμ.

micron in diameter in the case of psittacosis virus, or "parrot fever", down to about ten millimicrons for foot-and-mouth disease and poliomyelitis viruses. Put in another way, we may say that the diameter of virus particles varies from 250 millionths down to 10 millionths of a millimetre and that the smallest viruses have particles only some two or three times the diameter of a haemoglobin molecule.

If we consider the larger viruses, in the first place we are led almost inevitably to the conclusion that these viruses are very small bacteria with strict parasitic habits. As is shown in the table, the viruses and the free-living organisms overlap as regards size and it is impossible to draw a hard line between viruses on the one hand, and bacteria on the other; psittacosis virus elements are larger than the small sewage organisms, which are free living and non-pathogenic. Vaccinia virus elements are about the same size as those of the infective agents of agalactia of goats and pleuropneumonia of cattle. We know therefore that there is still room in a particle with a diameter of about 150 mμ. for that complex organisation which is necessary for an independent existence, including growth and multiplication.

As we have seen, vaccinia infection is always associated with small refractile granules which can be seen under dark-ground illumination, photographed with ultraviolet light, and stained by methods which load the particle heavily with dye. The more these "Paschen bodies", "elementary bodies" or "coccoid bodies" are studied, the more closely they are found to resemble many bacteria. They are constantly present, in very large numbers, in infective material such as raw calf-lymph or cultures in tissues, and they increase in numbers progressively with the disease. The elementary bodies may be purified by filtration, which removes cell fragments from a crude virus suspension, followed by centrifugation, which deposits the elementary bodies and frees them from soluble constituents or the original emulsion. The deposited particles may be washed and infectivity remains associated with the particles. Rivers and Ward have shown that, under the most favourable conditions, the number of particles is a fair measure of the infectivity of a virus suspension, and if all elementary bodies are removed the infectivity disappears. On morphological grounds, then, we must conclude that the "coccoid bodies" are the infective units of the virus, and to this extent they are homologous with the visible bacteria. But there is much more than this, for the elementary bodies behave to specific antisera in much the

(33)

same way as ordinary bacteria respond to their antisera. The virus may be neutralised by suitable doses of appropriate antisera, and such sera may be shown to clump or agglutinate the virus particles just as bacteria may be agglutinated by their specific antisera. Reactions between virus suspensions and antisera lead to the fixation of complement, and from crude virus suspensions (Smith) or from the virus bodies themselves (Cragie) it is possible to prepare a substance which, though not itself infective, gives specific precipitates with immune serum, and this is comparable with a bacterial haptene. As shown by M. H. Salaman, the virus neutralising element and the agglutinating constituent may be adsorbed and removed from an immune serum by means of purified "elementary bodies". All the serological reactions of vaccinia virus are found to have parallels in the interaction between bacteria and their antisera. Analysis of virus particles, as shown by Rivers and others, discloses the presence of proteins, fats and carbohydrates. In this respect again the elementary bodies are similar to bacteria, and other living organisms. Almost everything seems to agree with the view that vaccinia is a very small microorganism except for two things. (1) The purified virus bodies have never been shown to have any metabolism. (2) Vaccinia has not yet been grown apart from living cells. There are several explanations which might be tendered to explain these two difficulties. Like all viruses vaccinia is a strict intracellular parasite and it has been suggested that viruses will only grow inside cells, because it is only in that situation that they find some intermediate product of the host's cell metabolism on which they live. It may be pointed out that the leprosy bacillus has not yet been cultivated on artificial media, nor has it been shown to have an independent metabolism, but no one would class this relatively large organism with the viruses. On the whole the balance of evidence is strongly in favour of the view that vaccinia virus is a very small pathogenic micro-organism with strict parasitic habits.

If we consider some other larger members of the virus group, again we find there are many analogies with visible bacteria. The studies of Bedson and Bland, as also of Levinthal, show that the virus bodies of psittacosis, which can be stained, are strongly reminiscent of bacteria; their presence, whether in infected animals or in tissue cultures, is always associated with infectivity. They multiply progressively with the development of the disease and are absent from normal animals.

Serological studies with this virus are not so numerous or extensive as is the case with vaccinia virus, and for some unknown reason potent antisera are more difficult to prepare in this instance; yet such serological information as we possess (Bedson) harmonises with the view that the coccoid bodies represent small organisms.

Rivers and Ward have shown that, in the case of infectious myxomatosis of rabbits, the preparation of purified "elementary bodies" is practicable and that these behave both morphologically and serologically like minute organisms.

As we pass down the series of representative viruses to the smaller forms, accurate information becomes more scanty, yet suggestive observations may be found. Ledingham and Gye, for example, record that it is possible to centrifuge down small particles from filtrates which will induce tumours in fowls and ducks, to wash these particles with saline without materially impairing their infectivity, to make suspensions of the particles and to show that they are specifically agglutinated by antisera which neutralise the tumour-inducing agent. The infective units of the Rous sarcoma virus have diameters of only 75 mμ. and this small size makes studies of this kind very difficult, but the evidence, though admittedly scanty, is suggestive.

Now, although a good case can be made out for regarding the larger viruses as very small bacteria with parasitic habits, it becomes more and more difficult to imagine that the smallest representatives of the group can be regarded in the same way. In the case of foot-and-mouth disease, poliomyelitis and some of the bacteriophages, for example, it does not seem possible that there is room in a particle smaller than a molecule of haemocyanin and only two or three times the diameter of a haemoglobin molecule for the complexes necessary for organised life. So that for some years there have been those who regarded viruses as chemical substances which, having gained access to a cell, disturbed the normal metabolism of the host and induced in some way the formation of further quantities of the specific substance. Bordet, for example, regards bacteriophage as a chemical substance which on lysis of affected bacteria causes the production of more bacteriophage, and he has drawn analogies with the progressive production of fibrin ferment which occurs when fibrinogen is converted into fibrin.

The chemical theory of viruses received an immense stimulus from the work of Stanley in America when he announced "the isolation from diseased tobacco plants of a crystalline protein

possessing the properties of tobacco mosaic virus".
Stanley's protein does not occur in normal tobacco
plants, but develops in astonishingly large quantities in the plants after infection. The expressed
juice from a diseased plant may contain about ten
times as much soluble protein as a normal plant
and about 80 per cent of this total protein is the
abnormal constituent. The new protein is not
confined to the tobacco plant but appears in every
host plant that the virus can actively infect—even
in hosts in no way related to the tobacco plant,
such as spinach. Stanley's original claims, naturally
enough, met with much criticism and his work
has been repeated and extended by others. It may
fairly be said that although the original views have
been modified in certain particulars and purer
products than Stanley's original ones have been
obtained, the newer knowledge has not destroyed
Stanley's claim that the protein possessed the
properties of the virus, but rather strengthened it.
Bernal has shown, for example, that the crystals
are not true crystals but are more properly called
fibres or para-crystals, having two-dimensional
instead of three-dimensional regularity. X-ray
studies of highly purified preparations made by
Bawden and Pirie show that "the particles of the
virus are practically identical and pack together in

(38)

regular two-dimensional bundles". X-ray studies further "show unequivocally that regularities occur inside the particles" and "if there is any more 'vital' material about, it must be represented by only a small fraction of the bulk of the particles". Chemical and physical examinations have thus shown that the virus protein can be obtained in a very pure form and it is infective for tobacco plants in doses of about one ten thousand millionth of a gramme.

Bawden and Pirie have also extended the work and isolated proteins of similar type from three strains of tobacco mosaic and from two strains of cucumber mosaic which have serological affinities with tobacco mosaic. The five diseases caused by these viruses are all clinically different, and the corresponding proteins are distinct. They have further evidence that potato virus "X" is associated with another analogous but quite distinct protein. From tomato plants infected with the virus causing "bushy-stunt" these two workers have isolated a specific protein which crystallises in the form of rhombic dodecahedra, and there is therefore now one virus which can be isolated in the form of true crystals.

There is thus a solid body of evidence accumulating to show that some of the plant viruses are nucleo-proteins of unusual type with a very large molecular weight. The infective units in the sap of tobacco plants infected with mosaic disease can be filtered through membranes with an average pore-size of 53 mμ., but as the infective agent is purified and concentrated it becomes increasingly difficult to filter and the highly purified product will not pass through membranes with pores of 450 mμ. It appears, therefore, that on purification the original small elements in the infected sap aggregate into larger masses which are probably rod-shaped. It is not possible to be certain that virus and protein are one and the same, because it is impossible to be sure that protein preparations of this type are 100 per cent pure. It is admitted that the purest preparations of the protein so far obtained may contain a small percentage of impurity, but the amount of impurity is certainly very small. If we argue that it is possible that the Stanley protein owes its activity to the admixture of virus in small amounts with a high proportion of a strange protein—conceivably a primitive antibody produced by the plant—we are still faced with the difficulty that the infective element in the plant sap is of such small diameter (25 mμ.) that it is difficult to imagine it as a living organised structure. The balance of evidence is strongly in favour of the view that certain plant viruses are nucleo-proteins.

Stanley's results and the amplifications by others have made a profound impression on current thought regarding the nature of viruses, and several workers have attempted to show that mammalian viruses are heavy proteins similar to the virus proteins of plants. It must be confessed that the evidence for the chemical nature of mammalian viruses is, as yet, quite unconvincing. As we have seen it is possible to isolate and purify infective particles from crude virus emulsions by filtration, centrifugation and washing. In many instances a suspension of particles of fairly uniform size may be obtained which are infective and give reactions for proteins, but there is no evidence that the particles are even approximately pure protein, and this has been shown in the case of the plant viruses. It need hardly be pointed out that any minute organised cell might show these characters, and we know that vaccinia virus elementary bodies give reactions not only for proteins but also for fats and carbohydrates. The plant viruses which have yielded such remarkably interesting results are exceptionally favourable objects for study, for they can be obtained in large amount; they are remarkably stable substances and withstand chemical treatment and other insults which will destroy many other plant viruses and most of the mammalian ones. The study of mammalian viruses from this point of view is still in its infancy and it is possible that more significant and decisive advance will be made in the future.

Purified and concentrated preparations of bacteriophage have been prepared by Schlesinger and others, while more recently Northrop, as a result of his studies of such preparations, has propounded the view that bacteriophage, and probably by analogy other viruses, are "auto-catalytic proteins", forming more of themselves by some relatively simple ferment action from some preformed host constituent. Analogies are drawn with the formation of much trypsin from a little trypsin and a large supply of trypsinogen, or pepsin from pepsinogen, much as Bordet had used the analogy of fibrin ferment to explain his conception of bacteriophage. Stanley also considers that the proteins he isolated may be "auto-catalytic proteins". These theories of viruses presuppose that there is some constituent of the host's cell which can readily be transformed into virus, and that the normal cell builds up complexes from which viruses can be made by ferment action of the virus itself.

There are a number of serious difficulties in the way of accepting this view, even when it is proved that most viruses are pure proteins. If we consider the very large number of bacteriophages or viruses which can infect any one species, we have to postulate the formation of a correspondingly large number of precursors in the host, and no suggestion is ever made as to the function of the precursors in the host's normal economy. They can hardly be made just in order that virus diseases may develop. Again, if viruses arose in this way, the same precursor must exist in widely different species. The precursor of yellow fever virus must exist in man, mice, rhesus monkeys and a limited number of species of mosquitoes. The chorio-allantoic membrane of the developing egg in the case of the duck and the hen must contain precursors which do not exist in the hatched bird, for we know that these egg membranes will accept and nourish many viruses which the fully developed chick rejects.

If the formation of the virus from its precursor was a simple and easy matter, and the parent substance was a normal constituent of the body cells, we should expect viruses to arise spontaneously from time to time in isolated communities. There is, however, no evidence that they are ever created anew in this way. Bacterial cultures can be kept free from bacteriophage indefinitely with a little trouble. Great Britain is free from rabies as long as the quarantine laws are faithfully observed, outbreaks only occur when quarantine regulations are contravened. India has a large human and susceptible monkey population and the usual vector for yellow fever. For very many years, at any rate, there has not been an outbreak of yellow fever there; but great uneasiness is felt in certain quarters lest some day an infected mosquito should be transported to India in an aeroplane and thus start a disastrous epidemic in what would be for the yellow fever virus a virgin soil. There is, as yet, no good evidence that viruses ever arise *de novo* in a normal host, and there is much to indicate that they are always introduced from without.

Again, the viruses show well-developed antigenic characteristics and in many cases the host makes very potent antisera to the virus. This is readily intelligible if the virus is a foreigner, with an alien antigenic architecture, introduced from without, but it is much more difficult to explain if the virus arises by any simple ferment process from some preformed constituent of the host's cells.

The recent work on plant viruses and Stanley's heavy proteins supports the view that the virus is introduced from without. All workers stress the point that the heavy protein is a new substance foreign to the host and that it remains the same though the host be varied. Antigenically the virus protein is quite distinct from the proteins of the plant. It is very difficult to see how this new substance can be formed in such astonishingly large amount from the host's cells by any simple ferment action. The "auto-catalytic protein" view of viruses in its simplest form must therefore be rejected as unsatisfactory at the present time.

In our rapid review of the series of representative viruses it would seem that some of the smaller viruses are nucleo-proteins and that some of the larger viruses are parasitic micro-organisms. If we accept both sets of evidence, we reach the conclusion that the viruses are a heterogeneous collection of diverse agents which happen to induce disease states showing broad similarities. Blind acceptance of this view may make for peace and quietness, but it does not account for the common features met with in the group and ignores the remarkable gradation which exists between the largest and the smallest viruses. For example, vesicular stomatitis virus produces a disease which is very similar clinically to foot-and-mouth disease. so similar, indeed, are the two diseases that differential diagnosis is usually impossible for the clinician and appeal must be made to laboratory experiments to decide which infective agent is causing the disease. Foot-and-mouth disease virus is one of the smallest viruses (10 mμ. in diameter) and that of vesicular stomatitis is intermediate in size (85 mμ. in diameter). If we regard foot-and-mouth disease virus as a chemical substance and vaccinia virus (150 mμ.) as a micro-organism, how should we classify vesicular stomatitis virus? One cannot help feeling that there must be some factors common to the whole group, and we have either to attempt to reconcile the two opposing theories or adopt a non-committal attitude for the time being. Before closing I should like to put before you some speculations which lead me to the conclusion that it is possible to reconcile the two divergent views. Though direct evidence on the theory I propound is lacking, it appears to open up new lines of approach and to emphasise the importance of virus studies for all biologists.

All viruses are, as we have seen, specialised parasites and appear to be inanimate apart from living cells which they can infect. In many cases they can only multiply in certain hosts in which they often show preference for particular types of cells. They are thus probably some of the most highly specialised parasites in existence. The work of Fildes and his co-workers, Knight and Richardson, on the "factors" necessary for the growth of certain pathogenic bacteria has shown that with the development of the parasitic habit many bacteria may lose their power to synthesise substances essential for growth and multiplication; some, for example, lose the power to make an amino-acid and rely on the host to provide the missing essential substance. Certain strains of typhoid bacilli, for instance, require to be supplied with preformed tryptophane. A lost power of this kind can be regained under certain circumstances. Other organisms, such as staphylococci, may require nicotinic acid or its amide and aneurin (vitamin B_1). Others again, such as *Clostridium sporogenes*, require a factor which has not yet been accurately defined but which many other bacteria can synthesise for themselves. Parasitism has made the bacteria lazy. As Fildes puts it: "The parasitic bacteria have lost their power of synthesis owing to a persistent localisation in an environment where their 'factors' are preformed."

Lwoff has shown that haematin is necessary for certain protozoa, just as it is necessary for certain members of the haemophilus group of bacteria, and that the "V" factor required by this group is identical with pyridine-nucleotide-phosphate (Warburg's co-enzyme). In the absence of haematin and "V" factor the influenza bacillus will not grow. In nature both of these factors are provided by the host.

Mrs Pirie has recently shown that one of the small sewage organisms isolated by Elford and myself will take up oxygen and destroy glucose if the ferment catalase is present in the medium surrounding the organism. Without catalase, or else a relatively high concentration of haematin, oxidation of glucose cannot continue. It should be particularly noted that it is not necessary for the ferment to be taken up by the organism and built into the minute cell, as appears to be the case with the other bacterial factors we have been considering. The presence of catalase in the environment is all this tiny organism requires.

There is then much evidence to show that parasites through indolence give up making substances which are always at hand in the host's cells. The substances they filch from the host may be relatively simple substances, such as amino-acids, or more complex, such as co-ferments, and, as we have seen, a highly complex ferment in the medium surrounding an organism of virus size may have a profound influence on its metabolism. Apply this information to the group of very highly specialised parasites—the viruses, follow the indications to the limit, and we can form a possible explanation for the whole series, from micro-organism to molecule. We would suppose that the larger viruses were organisms which had lost the power to synthesise some factor or factors essential for their growth and multiplication, perhaps a ferment and co-ferments. As we pass down the scale and the viruses diminish in size, we would postulate the loss of more and more factors essential for growth. The intermediate sized viruses would have lost several essential ferment systems, and if we carry the suggested process to its logical conclusion we would find that the smallest viruses would have lost all ferments and all auto-synthetic potentialities. The diminution in size may in fact be a rough measure of the number of ferment systems lost. Divorced from the particular cells which they can infect, the structures we postulate would be inert and in a state of suspended animation; within the correct cell, however, they would have at hand all substances required for growth, and they would attract to themselves the requisite ferment systems from the host cells or utilise those in their immediate neighbourhood. They would, as it were, live a borrowed life, truly the supreme summit of parasitism. It may be suggested, in passing, that the cellular damage the viruses cause may be in large measure due to the deviation of essential substances and ferments from their normal function in the host's cells. We are still very ignorant of the details of the methods by which viruses poison their hosts. The one thing the perfect parasite possessed of its very own would be the chemical substance which transmitted the characters of the species, for it is an outstanding fact that the majority of viruses breed true. Many can be propagated through quite a number of different species for many generations and their essential characters remain unchanged. If the view I have just outlined receives favourable consideration, it would mean that, in the case of some of the plant viruses, at any rate, we appear to be within sight of a biochemical study of the nucleoproteins which transmit the character of a species. Truly this is a fascinating subject for the biochemist of to-day and to-morrow.

This view that viruses are decadent forms of organisms degraded through long persistent parasitism will, I think, appeal to many, even if they are not prepared to go the whole distance along the path I have outlined. Yet the view put forward gives a possible explanation for the whole series, the absence of any clean-cut separation between the smallest free-living organisms and the larger viruses, and all the gradations we encounter within the group. It also indicates how viruses probably arose, and explains their remarkable specificity. Dale, in the Huxley Lecture 1935, presented the arguments for and against the origin of viruses by heterogenesis, and concluded at that date that the biogenetic origin of the viruses was the more probable. The conclusion was based partly on the evidence submitted but more on the fact that whenever, in the past, biogenesis had been on trial it ultimately emerged triumphant. In agreement with this view I have ventured to speculate and put forward a theory of the origin of viruses.

Speculations and theories of this kind are of more value when they lead to progress, and, if there is any truth in the view put forward, Nature has presented us with a whole series of forms of life passing by fine gradations from a complete organism capable of independent existence down to the irreducible minimum required to transmit the characters of the species. Intensive study in such a series cannot fail to give fundamental information regarding vital processes of supreme interest alike to the biochemist as to all biologists. If the theory is wholly incorrect, work on these lines will not be wasted, for it is abundantly evident that a proper understanding of virus diseases and viruses is essential for the future well-being of mankind.

Milton Keynes UK
Ingram Content Group UK Ltd.
UKHW020111171024
449665UK00008B/76